- LINES TO LIVE BY -

# ARIANA GRANDE

Say 'thank you, next' to the bad vibes
and live your best life

POP PRESS

1

Published in 2022 by Pop Press, an imprint of Ebury Publishing,
20 Vauxhall Bridge Road,
London SW1V 2SA

Pop Press is part of the Penguin Random House group of companies
whose addresses can be found at global.penguinrandomhouse.com

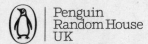

Penguin
Random House
UK

Copyright © Pop Press 2022
Illustrations © Pop Press 2022

First published by Pop Press in 2022

www.penguin.co.uk

A CIP catalogue record for this book is available from the British Library

Design: Seagull Design
Text: Charlotte Cole
Illustrations: LJG Designs

ISBN 9781529149388

Printed and bound in Great Britain by Clays Ltd, Elcograf S.p.A.

The authorised representative in the EEA is Penguin Random House Ireland,
Morrison Chambers, 32 Nassau Street, Dublin D02 YH68

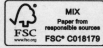

# CONTENTS

# ARI'S LINES
# TO LIVE BY

Ari is slaying it.

Several albums in, Ariana Grande has won numerous awards, and she kills it with her amazing vocal range and cute sense of style. She's a badass creative genius and fearless businesswoman – but she also knows when to step back and take time out for herself.

This book is packed with Ariana's wisdom and the lines that she lives by. If you need a dose of confidence or resilience. If you need advice on love or friendship, or want to know which fierce women inspire Ari's life. If you want to get empowered to challenge misogyny, get creative, or find out what success really means, then this is the place for you.

Whatever kind of empowerment you need or inspiration you're looking for, it's time to say thank you, next, to the bad vibes, put your bunny ears on and take the world by storm the Ariana Grande way.

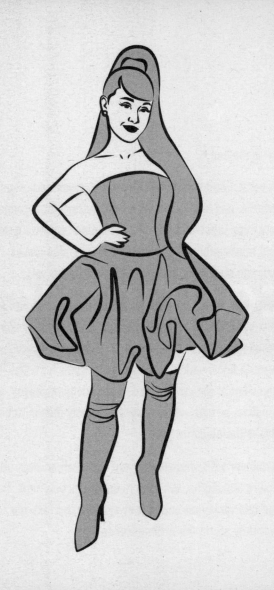

# CONFIDENCE

'I am going to spend
my time being the best
at what I do and not
worrying about what
people will think of it.'

'I have to be careful, but I would say that what you see is what you get, I'm pretty honest, I'm pretty authentic. I try to keep it real, because who the f*ck cares?'

'Sometimes people can confuse my niceness for weakness – or ditziness or stupidity. But it doesn't go hand-in-hand in that way, you know what I mean?'

'Of course I have to respect what everyone has to say, but I also have to follow my heart.'

'It took me a while to come into my own, to be unafraid, to be myself and to just be unapologetically honest, and that's a brave thing, that's a dangerous thing.'

'If things happen that you need to stand up for yourself for, you absolutely should take the opportunity.'

'I would rather sell
fewer records and
be outspoken.'

'Being yourself is one of the coolest things that you can do. As hard as it may be to get there, once you find that comfort, run with it.'

'I feel I'm at a point where I can use my voice and I can yell about things I'm passionate about, and that's a blessing.'

'#hashtag zerof*cks'

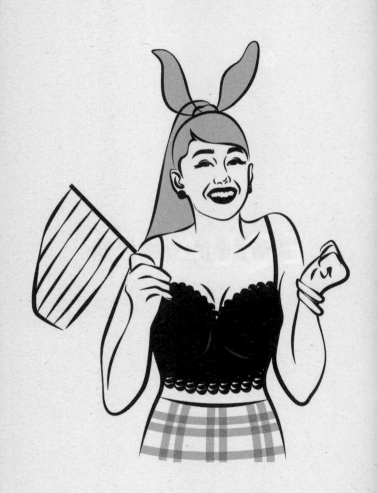

# EQUALITY

'Women should be able to express themselves however they like. I think that's feminism.
Taking pride in your body. Taking pride in your work. Doing whatever you want.'

'There's so much comparison for girls in this industry, it's just ridiculous.'

'Misogyny is ever-present, and we have to be there to support one another. That's really it. It's about the sisterhood. There's no competing in that. We have to lift each other up, not try and claw each other down.'

'I think I feel the pressure to respond [to sexism] not because I'm reacting to a personal attack, but because I feel like I want to fight for everyone.'

'Intolerance, meanness, double standards, misogyny, racism, sexism. All that sh*t. There's lots that we've got to start on. That's what we need to focus on. We've got work to do.'

'When a young male artist posts a shirtless picture on Instagram the comments will be like "Oh my God, heart eyes, so hot, babe alert!" [ . . . ] If a woman posts a suggestive photo or anything that expresses her own sexuality or confidence within her body, it's a very different response.'

'I'll never be able to swallow the fact that people feel the need to attach a successful woman to a man when they say her name.'

'I'm not Big Shaun's ex.
I'm not Niles's possible
new girl. I'm Ariana
Grande and if that's not
interesting enough,
don't talk to me.'

'How are we going to get this right for a country that is made up of so many different, diverse beautiful people if the whole sh*t is being run by straight white old men?'

'We're in such a trying time and people have been responding with acceptance, love, inclusion and passion [ . . . ] This generation, they're standing up and they're not going to take no for an answer.'

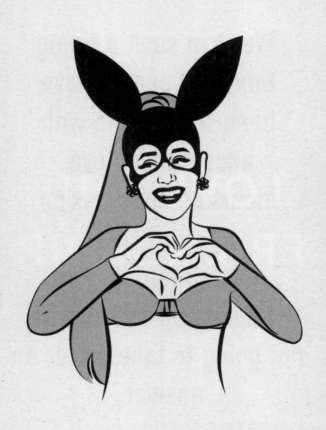

# LOVE AND FRIENDSHIP

'Having your heart broken is awful but you have two choices: you can sulk or you can choose to remain positive. Stay positive that you'll fall in love again.'

'A lot of empowered and strong people will be afraid to fall in love or be in a relationship because they think it will take away from their independence. [ . . . But] that is independence, because it's a choice to fall in love with someone.'

'There isn't a certain kind of beauty that I look for or appreciate or one thing [that] is more beautiful than the other. I love people's uniqueness. I love the quirky, weird and interesting – different things about everybody.'

'Love comes in many different forms. You can love somebody and not be in love with them. They can break your heart and you can cry over it but still not be in love with them. Love is a really peculiar thing.'

'Everybody has certain things that make them feel insecure. [ . . . ] But I feel like I'm at a point in my life where love is the most important thing, and I won't let anything come before it.'

'I have a bunch of really dope friends I've known since elementary school [ . . . ] They're going to keep me healthy and humble.'

'We're not big partiers, my friends and I, we're really sort of like nerds.'

'If other people are asking me to do things I'm uncomfortable with I just won't be friends with them.'

'I'm looking forward to hopefully learning to give some of the love and forgiveness that I've given away so frivolously and easily to men in the past to myself.'

'I'm so happy – that's all
I want, is to be with my
friends and family.'

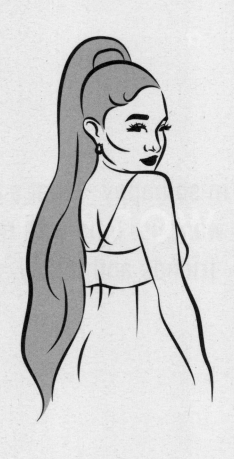

# WORK IT

'When you're handed a challenge [ . . . ] instead of sitting there and complaining about it, why not try to make something beautiful?'

'This is what I love to do and I will do it, is the mentality that my family kind of has.'

'For me, music has come first and foremost [ . . . ] I only care about becoming better at my craft and creating and writing and expressing myself.'

'I do have a lot to say and I do enjoy talking to people and I do want to do interviews and share with people and not be afraid to be myself.'

'I like to immediately start thinking about, what's next?'

'I love working. I get a day off and I'm confused.'

'[I'm] the biggest perfectionist you've ever met in your entire life.'

'I want my music to be as good as possible, so I'm open to hearing everybody's opinion. That doesn't mean I'm going to agree with it, but I'm very open to having help and constructive criticism and collaborating.'

'[My career is] much more work than anyone could ever imagine, but it's definitely worth it because I'm getting to do what I love.'

'Always listen to yourself
[ . . . ] don't listen to
outside sources
telling you what you
should be if you know
deep down if it's correct
or not.'

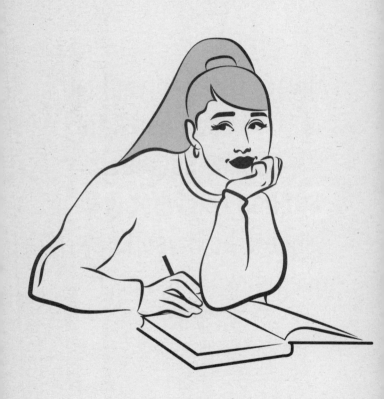

# CREATIVITY

'I'm all about the art. I just like to make music.'

'Music is the thing that
makes people feel good.
It's the thing that speaks
most to people's spirits
and we just wanted
to lift them.'

'It's exciting to change
it up.'

'[Music] is a great form of self-expression, I love it. It's nerve-wracking, but it's what I want to do.'

'If I'm not writing about
what I'm directly feeling
and what I'm going
through in this moment as
honestly and as genuinely
as I can, then I'm gonna
feel like I'm sacrificing
my artistry.'

'Just, like, experiment and have fun.'

'My favourite part of the music-making process is right when you finish a new song and you [ . . . ] put it in the car and listen to it on the way home really loud, and that's the most exciting part.'

'I just try to make music
that makes me happy,
that I'm most
passionate about.'

'When I'm writing I write directly about my life.'

'I think you just have to listen to what's inside [ . . . ] I think I've kind of learnt that the more authentic and genuine it is, the better it will work for you.'

'I would be compromising my artistry if I didn't keep it honest and true to what I'm going through.'

'I was like, whatever, let's do it and have some fun.'

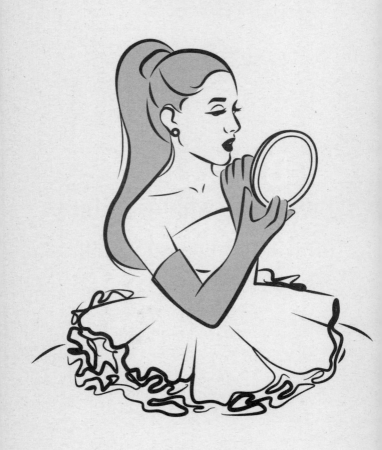

# BEAUTY
# AND
# FASHION

# 'I'm clearly a girly girl.'

'I think that fashion should be more of a self-expression thing as opposed to a trend thing. To me, when I feel really dope and I have an outfit on that makes me really happy, that's so much better.'

'I love an animal ear, clearly [ . . . ] I actually fell asleep in them last night, I'm not going to lie. They're just fun.'

*More* on why Ari wears
cat ears:

'I just like them.'

'As far as heels go, comfort is never part of the question.'

'Sometimes I have to shop
for myself with my mom
and just do it that way.'

'Even when I get my makeup done professionally I always like to do my liner because it's fun and feels good.'

'Every time I put my hair up, it's like a surprise. I forget how much I love it, and then I tie it back and I'm like, "I love this look! Ooh, girl!" Every time I tie it up is like the first time. It's true love.'

'Sometimes it can be hard to be yourself in a world where there are such high standards, and people tell you you have to be a certain kind of beautiful. Or only one kind of body is being glorified in the media.'

'I think you can wear whatever you want. I think you can one day wear a conservative sort of pantsuit or whatever – cover up – and the next day you can wear a miniskirt and thigh-high boots if you want.'

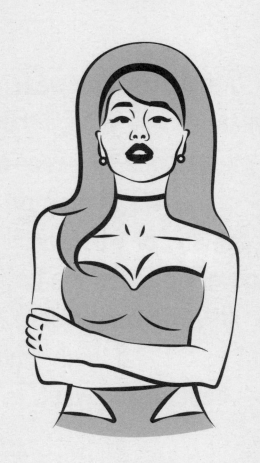

# MENTAL HEALTH

'Mental health is so important. People don't pay enough mind to it because we have things to do. [ . . . ] That's why I felt it was important, I just wanted to give people a hug, musically.'

'I wanted to break free
from all that I felt
was making me enjoy my
life a little less.'

'When I started to take care of myself more, then came balance, and freedom, and joy.'

About healing from anxiety:

'It takes hard work and practice and therapy and self-care. And so much love [ . . . ] It's just in your head and it's just so crazy how powerful it is.'

'Keep it grateful.
Keep it cute.'

'I think when we make each other feel safe or go the extra mile to be accepting or celebratory of other people, even if we aren't the same [ . . . ] that's going to help us get through this tough ass time together.'

'It has helped me deal with so much. I think it's great for everybody. [ . . . ] Therapy is the best. It really is.'

'Staying close to my family and my friends, that was really the most helpful to me [ . . . ] it puts things in perspective, it reminds me of what's real and what's sort of nonsense and not to be paid attention to.'

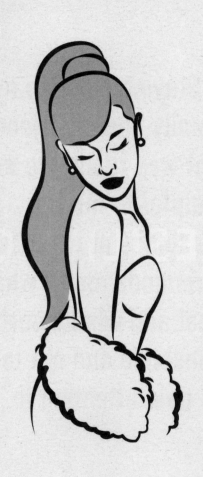

# RESILIENCE

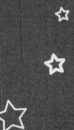

'Every time you read something that upsets you, just walk away and do something else.'

'I've done a really good job of deciding what matters to me, and if someone has a problem with me, like: "OK . . . truth is, you don't f*cking know me so [*shrugs*]" – it's OK.'

'I want to thank my nonna for [ . . . ] for teaching me to laugh off any negativity that tries to derail me and to have compassion for the haters.'

'I find rain very calming
and, like, peaceful.'

'Maybe I should be giving these chances to myself, instead of everybody else again and again and again, and that works for me personally and also [in] music.'

'If you're someone out there who has no idea what this next chapter's going to bring, you're not alone in that.'

'Regardless of what business you're involved in or what industry you work in, taking care of yourself is a full-time job.'

'I think that life is a process, and that everyone has their fair share of a tonne of sh*t on their plate, but we all work hard and deal with what we're dealing with, and we take each day at a time, and I'm happy.'

'I feel like I'm testing my limits. I feel like I'm coming into my own.'

'My fans know who I am, my family know who I am, my friends know who I am, and that's all that matters.'

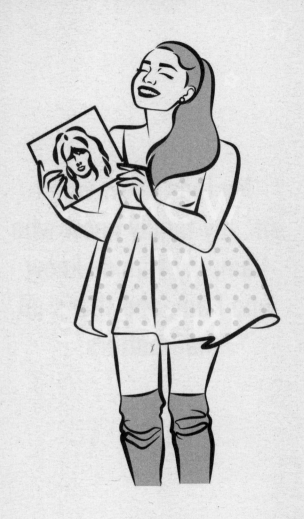

# WOMEN
# WHO
# INSPIRE

'My mom's a CEO, an engineer, a mom, the most fierce, badass b*tch in the world and I think I learn a lot of that from her, because she does everything herself as well.'

'My nonna actually got me started. My nonna took me for my first audition ever for *Annie* when I was eight. My nonna's wonderful.'

'She's paved the way for every female artist who's working today. Everyone who is in the pop game right now is doing something that Madonna probably did first.'

On Doja Cat:

'I love her personality. I love what she brings to the table musically. She's just such a breath of fresh air. I think she's brilliant and so talented.'

On Iggy Azalea in 'Problem':

'When you hear Iggy, it screams confidence and girl power, and all these wonderful things.'

'My all-time favourite artist is Imogen Heap. I'm in love with her, I'm obsessed with her. She's incredible, she's a genius and I've loved her forever.'

'I love Nicki [Minaj] so much. She kills it every single time. I love working with her as she's such a strong female and I think her punchlines are so great and her flow is so great. She's so talented.'

'Taylor Swift is an amazing songwriter. She's so relatable and so fun.'

On Judy Garland:

'I love how she tells a story when she sings. It was just about her voice and the words she was singing – no strings attached or silly hair or costumes, just a woman singing her heart out.'

'Whitney Houston is just my goddess, I love her so much [ . . . ] Rest in peace. She's just an angel.'

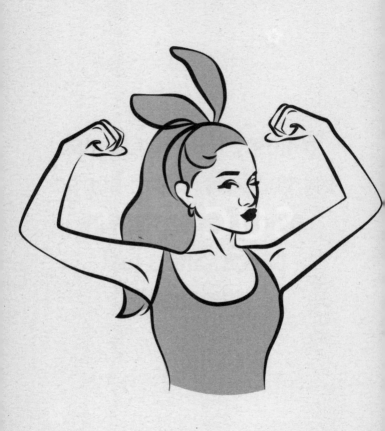

# SUCCESS

'I feel really blessed and
I'm not taking anything
for granted.'

'I think I'm still coming into my own. I think I'm still learning so much. I'm still growing so much.'

'I really haven't had a moment to just be still and really think about it. But I'm so lucky.'

'If you can be me for Halloween, if drag queens can dress up as me, then I'm a character. Go to your local drag bar, and you'll see it. That's, like, the best thing that's ever happened to me. It's better than winning a Grammy.'

'I want people to remember how I made them feel they weren't alone. And I want people to feel empowered and like they can get through things. [ . . . ] I want to make people feel strong.'

'Music means so much to me, so the fact that people are being so nice about it and responding so well to me, makes me the happiest girl in the world.'

'It's not about comparing myself to other people's success. I wanna celebrate what I'm doing, and I think that's special.'

'I just try to make music that makes me happy. That is what I am passionate about. I don't really pay attention to the celebrity part of it all. I only care about the music.'

'I like to laugh at myself, if you can't laugh at yourself then you can't live a proper life.'

'I don't like to worry too
much about the future,
I don't like to think too
much about the past,
I like to just enjoy what's
happening now.'

'The more honest you are and f*cks less you give, it really might turn out to be a beautiful thing for you.'

'My momma [taught me] to work hard, give generously, and that behind every successful woman is herself.'

# ACKNOWLEDGEMENTS

P2 from coupdemainmagazine.com, 'Ariana Grande on her loves, problem-solving and her new album' (2014), P3 from papermag.com, 'In Conversation: Troye Sivan and Ariana Grande' (2018), P4 from Time.com, 'Ariana Grande: I Do Not Always Order a Grande from Starbucks' (2014), P5 from flavourmag.co.uk, 'Interview with Yours Truly, Ariana Grande!' (2013), P6 from interview on *Music Choice HD* (2017), P7 from On Demand Entertainment, 'Ariana Grande interview: Sam and Cat star talks dating tips, boybands, music and Miley Cyrus' (2013), P8 from Vogue.com, 'Ariana Grande on Grief and Growing Up' (2019), P9 from Byrdie.com, 'Ariana Grande Shares Her #1 Beauty Tip (and It's Not What You'd Expect)' (2020), P10 From the *Zach Sang Show* (2015), P11 from Vogue, '73 Questions with Ariana Grande' (2020), P14 from Fairfax Media interview (2014), P15 from Power 106 Los Angeles, *Big Boy's Neighborhood* (2013), P16 from Coveteur.com 'Ariana Grande Opens Up About Her Emotional Tour & Keeping A Healthy Perspective' (2017), P17 from BBC Radio 1Extra, *Breakfast* (2015), P18 from Power 106 Los Angeles, 'Ariana Grande Checks In With Eric D-Lux & Justin Credible' (2015), P19 from graziadaily.co.uk, 'Ariana Grande Goes Big On Her Female Activist Calling' (2016), P20 from billboard.com, 'Ariana Grande on Defending Female Pop Stars and Staying Away From Drama' (2016), P21 from *Honeymoon Diaries* (2015), P22 from *Zach Sang Show* (2020), 'Ariana Grande "Positions" Interview' (2020), P23 from heatworld.com, 'Ariana Grande found stable ground where there was none' (2018), P26 from dolly.com.au, 'Cover girl Ariana Grande chats music, florals and sparkles – and why she's not a fan of red carpets' (2014), P27 From *heatworld*, 'Ariana Grande speaks to James Barr for heat Radio!' (2016), P28 from Coveteur.com 'Ariana Grande Opens Up About Her Emotional Tour & Keeping A Healthy Perspective' (2017), P29 from Complex.com, 'Ariana Grande: "Shadow of a Doubt" ' (2013), P30 from Seventeen.com, 'Ariana Grande Reveals How She Beat Insecurity & Found *Huge* Success' (2014), P31 from billboard.com, 'Ariana Grande on Defending Female Pop Stars and Staying Away From Drama' (2016), P32 from 90.3 Amp Radio, *The Shoboy Show* (2016), P33 from TheHotDeskTV, *Ariana @ The Hot Desk* (2014), P34 from acceptance speech, Billboard Woman of the Year Award (2018), P35 from *Ariana Grande Backstage at the B96 Pepsi Summer Bash* (2014), P38 from *Time*, 'Ariana Grande Is Ready to Be Happy' (2018), P39 from *Loose Women* (2015), P40 from *Ariana Grande's Full Interview with Shazam top 20* (2014), P41 from *Entertainment Tonight, Ariana Grande Fights Back TEARS Defending Herself Against 'Diva' Accusation* (2020), P42 from Apple Music, *Ariana Grande: 'Sweetener' Interview* (2018), P43 from British *Vogue, Waking Up with Ariana Grande* (2018), P44 from ClevverTV, *Ariana Grande Talks 'Yours Truly,' Tour & Fashion* (2013), P45 from AskAnythingChat (2013), P46 from Ariana Grande Interview, https://www.youtube.com/watch?v=QoWvuTabA4Y (2013), P47 from Billboard, *Ariana Grande Reacts to Being Woman of The Year, Talks Celebrating Women & More* (2018), P50 from Capital FM, 'Ariana Grande Grande Talks About Her Relationship With Nathan from The Wanted' (2013), P51 from *Entertainment Tonight, Ariana Grande Fights Back TEARS Defending Herself Against 'Diva' Accusation* (2020), P52 from MTV News, *Ariana Grande's interview with Gabby Wilson* (2016), P53 from the *Zach Sang Show*, 'EXCLUSIVE Interview with Ariana Grande' (2014), P54 from the *Zach Sang Show* (2015), P55 from Apple Music, *Ariana Grande: 'Sweetener' Interview* (2018), P56 from AskAnythingChat (2013), P57 from Billboard, Ariana Grande Answers Twitter Questions (2013), P58 from TheHotDeskTV, *Ariana @ The Hot Desk* (2014), P59 from British *Vogue, Waking Up with Ariana Grande* (2018), P60 from *Entertainment Tonight, Ariana Grande Reveals How Grandma Inspired Her Platinum 'Focus' Makeover* (2015), P61 from *Time*, 'Ariana Grande Is Fully Aware That the Lyrics of "Break Free" Make No Sense' (2014), P64 from Madoff Productions, Backstage Interview: Ariana Grande (2017), P65 from papermag.com, 'In Conversation: Troye Sivan and Ariana Grande' (2018), P66 from *Daily Mail*, ' "I love an animal ear": Ariana Grande ditches her style' (2018), P67 from Power 106 Los Angeles, 'Ariana Grande Says Why She Wears Cat Ears' (2014), P68 from 'An oceanUP Interview with Ariana Grande' (2011), P69 from ClevverTV, 'Ariana Grande Talks Music at the Creative Arts Emmy Awards 2011' (2011), P70 from GlamourMagazine.co.uk, 'Ariana Grande chats to GLAMOUR about her MAC Viva Glam collaboration' (2016), P71 from Byrdie.com, 'Ariana Grande Shares Her #1 Beauty Tip (and It's Not What You'd Expect)' (2020), P72 from *Good Morning America* (2015), P73 from *Loose Women* (2015), P76 from Apple Music, *Ariana Grande: Manchester and Mental Health* (2018), P77 from Time.com, 'Ariana Grande: I Do Not Always Order a Grande from Starbucks' (2014), P78 from *Time*, 'Ariana Grande Is Ready to Be Happy' (2018), P79 from *Ariana at the BBC* (2018), P80 & cover from *Zach Sang Show*, Ariana Grande "thank u, next" Interview (2019), P81 From KIIS-FM, 'Ariana Grande Reveals "Sweetener" Album, "The Light is Coming" Single at KIIS FM's Wango Tango' (2018), P82 from thefader.com, 'Ariana Grande found stable ground where there was none' (2018), P83 from *Today Show* (2014), P86 from coupdemainmagazine.com, 'Interview: Ariana Grande on her loves, problem-solving and her new album' (2014), P87 From AskAnythingChat (2013), P88 from acceptance speech, Billboard Women in Music Rising Star Award (2016), P89 From Z100 Radio (2013), P90 from *Zach Sang Show*, 'Ariana Grande "thank u, next" Interview (2019) – 6ᵗʰ P91 from acceptance speech, Billboard Woman of the Year Award (2018), P92 from Fairfax Media interview (2014), P93 from AskAnythingChat (2016), P94 from KIIS-FM, 'Ariana Grande Spills Tea on New Album Collabs + Answers Fan Questions', P95 from https://www.youtube.com/watch?v=eVS3MUb31Uk, P98 from *Zach Sang Show*, 'Ariana Grande "Positions" Interview' (2020), P99 from *Live with Kelly and Michael* (2015), P100 from *Good Morning America* (2018), P101 from Apple Music, *Ariana Grande: Justin Bieber Collaboration "Stuck With U" and Unreleased Doja Cat Song* (2020), P102 from Seventeen.com, 'Ariana Grande Reveals How She Beat Insecurity & Found *Huge* Success' (2014), P103 from *Jimmy Kimmel Live* (2016), P104 from KIIS-FM, 'Ariana Grande Spills Tea on New Album Collabs + Answers Fan Questions', P105 from ClevverTV, 'Ariana Grande Talks New Music' (2011), P106 from Billboard.com, 'Gimme Five: Ariana Grande's Most Inspirational Female Singers' (2013), P107 from Ariana Grande Interview, https://www.youtube.com/watch?v=QoWvuTabA4Y (2013), P110 from ClevverTV, 'Ariana Grande Talks Music at the Creative Arts Emmy Awards 2011' (2011), P111 from 90.3 Amp Radio, *The Shoboy Show* (2016), P112 from *Ariana at the BBC* (2018), P113 from Vogue.com, 'Ariana Grande on Grief and Growing Up' (2019), P114 from BBC Radio 1Extra, *Breakfast* (2015), P115 from flavourmag.co.uk, 'Interview with Yours Truly, Ariana Grande!' (2013), P116 from Hot 97, Ariana Grande: Sings, curses and talks kissing Mac Miller! (2013), P117 from dolly.com.au, 'Cover girl Ariana Grande chats music, florals and sparkles – and why she's not a fan of red carpets' (2014), P118 from *Rosso on Drive* (2014), P119 from *Zach Sang Show*, 'Ariana Grande "thank u, next" Interview' (2019), P120 from Billboard, *Ariana Grande Reacts to Being Woman of The Year, Talks Celebrating Women & More* (2018), P121 from acceptance speech, Billboard Women in Music Rising Star Award (2016)

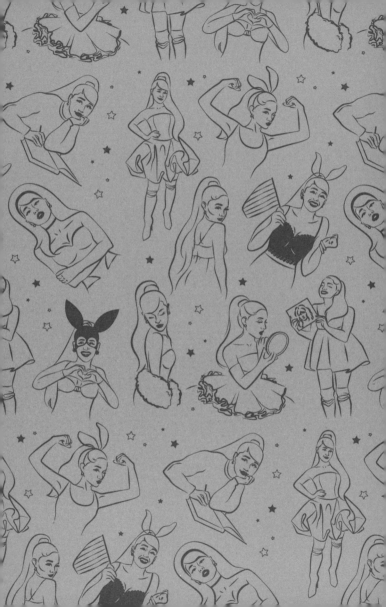